The Secret Natural Penis Enlargement Guide for Men

(How to Make Your Penis Bigger)

The Best Exercises, Tips, and Techniques for Enhancing Your Penis Girth and Length; Valuable Methods for Increasing Your Hardness; Increasing Your Capacity for Making Love; Increasing Your Ejaculation Control; and Much More...

Disclaimer

Copyright © by Daniel.J. miller 2023. All rights reserved.

Table of contents

Introduction

How to Begin

It's necessary to prepare yourself before starting any exercise or penis-extension technique. Ahead of time, make sure your penis is ready before you get into the action. ready to get the spotlight. The goal of doing this is to protect your penis throughout your interventions as well as to provide the best possible outcomes.

1. Soak a soft washcloth in a bowl of water that is just warm enough to be cozy but not painfully hot. To get a damp but not dripping-wet cloth, squeeze away the extra water.
2. Squeeze the towel tightly around the penis shaft. You can experiment to find which suits you best because it doesn't matter if you are hard or soft when you do this.
3. removing the cloth and soaking it in the water bowl once more after holding it in place for at least a minute. To wrap your penis three times in all, repeat the procedure twice.
4. Now that your penis is completely dry, you can start using it.

It is not just for cleaning purposes that you should apply a hot compress to your penis before starting your exercises. Your crotch will be drawing a lot of blood, which will improve the blood flow there and make the skin around it stretcher. Making your workouts as useful as possible is made possible by both of these factors.

And lastly, it will indeed have the advantage of wiping any sweat or dirt from your penis, which will help you acquire a nice, strong grip when you start exercising.

Option One: Stretching It

Stretching your length is the primary focus of your first set of workouts, which is more than adequate to move you closer to your ultimate objective. In addition to your penis, the erectile tissue will also be stretched.

Try out all four of the potential stretching exercises over the next few days to see which one suits you the best. You just need to choose one. Change to another one if any of them hurt you, are challenging for you to accomplish, or don't appear to be having the desired impact in your particular situation.

In fact, the first stretching exercise we'll cover is a very well-liked one and is the one that men cite as the key to their success most frequently.

Depending on what is most comfortable for you, you can either execute the exercise while standing up or while sitting down. Your penis should be flaccid when you start.

1. Firmly hold the head of your penis in one hand, being careful not to cut off the blood flow.
2. As far as you can without hurting yourself, and especially without hurting yourself, extend the head of your penis.
3. While counting the minutes on a timer, maintain it in place for five complete minutes. Pull the head of your penis a little bit further once each minute is complete. It's possible that doing this will make you uncomfortable, especially at the beginning of your penile augmentation program. If so, give up rather than continue to pull while endangering yourself. In order to stretch without experiencing discomfort, keep trying.

4. Give yourself a full minute of relaxation when the five minutes have passed.

5. Next, whip your penis around in a circular motion. At least 30 circular motions should be performed. It's crucial not to omit this because the goal is to reactivate any blood flow that may have been restricted during stretching.

6. Four more times, pull for five minutes, with a slight variation each time. Each time, choose a different direction to draw your penis in, such as upwards, downwards, or to the left or right. Throughout a session, avoid giving the same instructions more than once. By doing so, you'll be sure to extend your penis as effectively as possible while paying equal attention to each part of it. Repeat the whipping motions at least 30 times every five minutes.

7. Extend your penis as far as it will go in front of you for a full minute, always without pain or discomfort.

8. Tugging too hard will cause pain, so give your penis ten light pulls.

9. Once your penis has had a chance to rest, you are finished for the day. Repeat this exercise the next day.

Last but not least, you should try to avoid putting any pressure on the dorsal nerve, which runs down the top of your penis. You will undoubtedly experience pain and will be unable to profit from the activity as a result.

The men who have suggested this exercise assert that they noticed a difference after just two weeks and continued to experience improvements for up to four months after that, leading to many inches of growth.

Option Two: **Stretching It**

Although slightly less complex than the first stretching exercise, this one isn't really that different. If you're not yet confident in your technique or if the additional stretching required by Option 1 makes you uncomfortable, this can be a great place to start. Once more, in order to properly do this exercise, your penis must be flaccid. To do this, follow the preparatory instructions from the first chapter.

1. Take one hand and grab the penis' head. The same as always: your grasp shouldn't be painful but should still be firmly held.
2. Stretch the entire length of your penis by pulling it out in front of you.
3. Remain in this posture with your penis for 30 seconds, then release and take a few minutes to relax. Continue stretching until you have clocked up to 20 minutes, then stop for at least 20 minutes before starting again.
4. It is advisable to start this activity slowly. In the beginning, only stretch your penis for five minutes at a time; after that, gradually increase both the length of each session and the number of sessions you do throughout the day.

If you use this method carefully, you can achieve the same success as the men who have used it, who claim to have added up to two full inches to the length of their penis over time.

Neither your technique nor the additional stretching required by Option 1 will be pleasant for you. Again, to complete this exercise properly, your penis must be flaccid, so it's crucial to carry out the prior preparation that we discussed.

It was written about in the first chapter.

1. Take one of your hands and grasp the penis' head. As always, your grasp should be firm without being uncomfortable.
2. Extend your penis out in front of you so that you can feel the stretch throughout the entire length of its shaft.
3. After 30 seconds, keep your penis in this position; then, release it and take a few minutes to relax. Repeat as necessary until you've clocked up to 20 minutes of stretching, and then stop for at least 20 minutes before starting again.
4. It's better to start this activity off lightly. Start by stretching your penis for no more than five minutes at a time, and gradually increase both the length of each session and the number of sessions you do throughout the day.

Men who have used this method claim that it has gradually increased the length of their penis by up to two full inches; if you use it carefully, you can have the same success.

Option Three: **Stretching It**

The final exercise you could try involves stretching your penis both while it is erect and while it is flaccid. When you start, you want it to still be soft since the hard part will come later.

1. With your dominant hand, grab your penis and pull it away from your body. When you achieve a tugging motion, you will then let it return to its regular state.
2. Ten times through this stretch, hold it for roughly 15 to 20 seconds each.

3. Re-do step 1, but draw your penis at an angle to the right this time. Repeat the stretch, this time holding it for 15 to 20 seconds.

4. Carry out the procedure once more, but this time pull to the left.

5. Repetition number four involves pulling downward this time.

6. Your penis must be erect for the subsequent steps. To make this happen, gently rub the tip with your thumb.

7. Now, circle the very base of your penis with your dominant hand's thumb and fingers. Repeat this motion ten times while pulling forward about an inch. The idea is to push all the penile energy up toward the head.

8. Draw your penis to the right, spin it with your thumb and finger, and pull it outwards at the same time.

9. Follow the instructions from step 7, but this time drag your penis to the left rather than the right.

10. To finish the workout, slap your penis 10 times against each of your inner thighs while it is still upright and pulling outwards.

Option Four: Stretching it

This final option, which is the fourth, may be the best fit for you if you have a spiritual bent. It has spiritual components that you might or might not be familiar with and is based on old Taoist teachings. If so, this may seem like the obvious activity to help you improve your penis. If not, there is nothing stopping you from giving it a try nonetheless; you could find that it improves more than just your trouser bulge.

1. Take a deep breath in through your nose, down your throat, and then swallow to force the air all the way down into your stomach.

2. As the air you breathed in goes through your stomach and descends down your abdomen, keep pushing it lower until it reaches your penis.

3. At the same time, press your ball sack and anus together with the three middle fingers of one hand. The Taoist term for this is Hui-Yin. By doing this, you will concentrate all of your breath's force into your penis, where it will remain.

4. Your task there is finished; you may now resume your normal breathing rhythm.

5. In order to stretch your penis as much as you can without feeling pain, you will start pulling it back and forth at the same moment. Repeat this action 36 times, trying to keep your movements as rhythmic as you can.

6. Now stroke the head till you have an erection because you must continue with this workout with your penis erect.

7. Place your entire hand at the base of your penis and firmly slide it forward an inch. As a result of the breath energy you focused there, your penis will be forced upwards toward its head.

8. Pull your penis in the direction of the right, and then spin it 36 times in the direction of the clock.

9. repetition of the preceding action, but this time rotating your penis counterclockwise.

10. Lastly, lightly smack your penis 36 times against each of your thighs.

Although there is an additional step in this exercise compared to the third choice, it increases the force of your breath in the mixture. The Taoists think this will lengthen your penis, improve its tone, and—best of all—improve its function by allowing all the energy from your body and other organs to flow downward and into your penis.

The breathing exercise will enable you to unwind into the rhythmic movements and finish the workout, regardless of your spiritual beliefs or preference to avoid this kind of thinking.

"Use It or Lose It."

One thing you should always keep in mind as you work on your penile augmentation program is that the more you utilize your penis, the better condition it will be in. Doctors and researchers are aware of the fact that a penis's muscle can only remain toned and healthy if it receives frequent oxygen augmentation.

Fortunately, it's simple to accomplish this; all you have to do is force your penis to become erect on a frequent basis to stimulate the rush of blood that will provide the oxygen your penis needs.

Without consistent erections, your penis' tissue will begin to lose its suppleness, which is very negative for your

penile augmentation program. Your penis could eventually lose roughly an inch of length if it doesn't receive this regular oxygen infusion. That clearly goes against what you want to achieve, so make sure you're having lots of erections.

Don't worry if you experience erection problems during a certain time or location, such as when visiting your in-laws or when you are grieving. You simply need to ensure that you get enough sleep so that your penis can take care of itself if you let it. Your penis will harden when you are dreaming during the REM stage of sleep.

Your penis will perform enough of its own maintenance if you sleep for a length of time that allows for lots of REM cycles for it to avoid shrinking.

Working on width and length is great, but the ladies always seem to imply that your girth is what really matters. The circumference is something you should most definitely pay attention to if you want to improve your penis.

Fortunately, methods to increase your circumference have been used for many years, and people, civilizations, and tribes from all over the world and throughout history can attest to their efficacy. The secret is to exercise your penis while it is only slightly erect, as opposed to fully flaccid or erect.

This kind of workout is beneficial for the overall development of the penis, ensuring that its length and girth increase proportionally. Along the way, you'll also notice that the size and density of your penis increase. Jelqing, which means "milking" in Arabic, is what it's known as, and it's largely regarded as the greatest and most efficient natural way to increase the size of your penis. Men in regions like India, Africa, and the Middle East are reported to have finally grown their penises to an alarming 17 inches, despite not having those proportions at birth.

The methods are well-liked in the West as well, and most men who use them claim several inches of growth over the course of a year; one Californian man even quadrupled his penis size in that time.

The process involves forcing blood into your penis, which causes the gaps within to gradually expand in volume and become better able to contain blood while erect. In addition to growing its size and strength, you'll also be enhancing the health of your penis.

When performing milking activities, it's crucial to keep a few safety precautions in mind. For example, you should never conduct any of these exercises while you are completely erect.

Your penis's veins may suffer severe, possibly irreparable harm as a result of this.

If nothing else is specified, always use lubrication throughout these workouts. If you don't, you'll at best feel sore at the conclusion of the exercise, and at worst you might do permanent harm.

Developing Width: Shower Time

Before we begin your girth exercises, a brief overview of these techniques' history will familiarize you with their enduring appeal and the unique preparation that has always been employed to maximize their results. This ancient technique can be incorporated into your routine as well, and the outcomes are frequently hailed as fantastic.

Throw out your shower gel and choose the ancients' advice instead; you won't regret it.

Arabs, known for having large, powerful penises, have been known to engage in milking exercises for generations. A boy is only six years old when the work starts. A boy learns from his father that steadily stroking his penis would gradually increase its size and length by lengthening it from the base to the tip. He starts to perform this exercise in a ritualistic manner, devoting 30 minutes daily to it.

Wealthy lads are finally taken to a separate location, where they are stripped down by the attendant and given an oil massage on their penis. His muscles will all be relaxed, and his sexual stimulation will also be increased.

You might want to indulge in your own version of the oil blend to use while you are completing your enhancement program since it is thought to be the technique's secret component. You should start by standing close to a shower.

1. A heaping tablespoon of white or yellow corn meal mix and a quart of pure mayonnaise are all that are needed to form the combination.
2. Apply the oil mixture all over your body, beginning at your head and neck and working your way lower, while covering your hair with a shower cap. Down to your feet, cover your entire body.
3. While standing in the hot shower, avoid standing directly in the stream of water. You will benefit initially from the steam the shower is producing.
4. Slowly and deliberately, use circular motions to rub the mixture into your skin. To work on your face, if you'd like, you can use a cloth.
5. Adjust the temperature of the shower so that it is more comfortable, and let the water wash the oil mixture off your body. Your skin will start to tingle all over as you do this.

When your shower is finished, the results will be exquisite. You won't just be tingling; you'll also notice that your skin has a glow and satin sheen unlike anything you've ever seen, and you'll feel joyful and uplifted while remaining perfectly relaxed. When coupled with the milking movements we will discuss in the following chapter, this shower technique can be a great addition to your daily routine.

Developing Width, Option One

Your first option is a pretty straightforward approach that you should practice five days a week. The final outcome ought to be an improvement of up to three inches in girth, which increases proportionally with length. You should be aware that it's typical for guys who try this strategy to lose motivation within the first month because it's unlikely you'll experience any special results. But in the second month, you'll start to see just what you were looking for.

1. Lubricant should be applied to your penis, and it should be placed wherever you can quickly access it. You might need to add more lubricant during the activity.
2. Squeeze the base of your penis between your thumb and forefinger, pulling it up toward the tip while simultaneously pushing it downward. You should stop as soon as it starts to make your penis semi-erect, because that is the goal.

3. Always keep in mind that this exercise should never be done with the penis fully erected.

4. Form a circle with your thumb and forefinger, firmly grasp the base of your penis, and then pull in a long, continuous motion downward and outward.

5. Immediately put your other hand on the base of your penis and perform the motion again, this time going all the way through from the base to the tip.

6. Continue doing this while switching hands to produce a rhythmic milking motion. With the exception of the tip of the head, you should be moving your hands over the whole surface of your penis while remaining semi-rectilinear. Depending on what works best for you, if you start to feel totally tight, either stop for a time to let it pass or squeeze a little harder.

7. Continue until you have made 200 to 300 strokes with medium pressure, which should take about 10 minutes.

8. For the second week, gently increase the force of your strokes and keep going until you have completed between 300 and 500 strokes, which should take about 15 minutes.

9. Starting in the third week, you can do this exercise for 20 minutes every day, using as much pressure as you can bear without feeling pain to complete 500 strokes or more. If you need to, add additional lube, but never let your penis dry out because that will

cause a serious annoyance right where you'd rather not have it.

10.   After you're done, give your penis about 30 up-and-down slaps to let the blood flow there return to normal.

11.   This method is a serious test of self-control. It makes sense that when you rub your penis, your excitement will grow; after all, that is how it is supposed to work. You must halt or squeeze to prevent this so that you can finish the exercise while only partially upright.

Developing Width, Option Two

If it works for your approach, this method of milking is a terrific option because it is usually thought to have amazing impacts on width and total size. Again, before you start the workout, lubricate your penis and make sure you are just semi-erect at all times. If you are completely erect or soft, it won't work and may even be harmful.

1. With your penis semi-erect, rub a little extra lubricant between your palms and lubricant all over it.
2. Form a circle with your forefinger and thumb and firmly grasp the base of your penis. During the following phase, maintain this grasp.
3. Slide your hand all the way down to the head of your penis and simultaneously pull. Your penis's head will enlarge during the process, as you'll see.
4. Quickly perform the first two actions with your other hand.
5. Once the second hand has reached the top of your penis, switch back to the first. Continue doing this relatively quickly. If you find yourself approaching a climax, pause until the impulse passes once again.

Limit the number of repetitions you perform while milking to 200 in the first few weeks that you are training with this activity. It's vital to stop if you experience any pain or discomfort during this exercise, which should take about 10 minutes overall. If your penis is still sore, you should wait a few days before trying again. You can easily start again after a little break.

Start increasing the number of repetitions you include once you have been using this strategy for two complete weeks. At some point, you can spend up to 20 minutes and perform 400 repetitions in a single session.

Developing Width, Option Three

The third exercise to improve your penis' overall girth and strength is slightly different from the first two. You should be able to complete this exercise.

You should be aware that it will cause the head of your penis to expand more than you might anticipate and turn a very red hue, so you should be a little bit more gentle than you were while trying the others. You are forcing a lot of blood into the head of your penis, which is what will produce the color change. Don't worry; this is a typical reaction to the workout. Of course, there shouldn't be any pain involved at all, and you should stop immediately if there is.

1. While the penis is still soft, thoroughly apply lubrication to the shaft.
2. Extend your penis downward and to the side a little bit with your thumb and first finger.
3. Pull your penis to the other side and do it again with your other hand.
4. To mimic the motion of milking, keep repeating with one hand after the other. Start out gently, but once

you're halfway there, you can start using more force while still being mild.

For the first several days, repeat the procedure 100 times. Then, start gradually increasing the repetitions each day. You should eventually be able to perform 200 repetitions painlessly.

Developing Width, Option Four

Men who desire to enlarge the head of their penis are the target audience for this method. It is much the same as the first strategy you used to increase your circumference, but much more slowly and gently. The Tao technique is one name for it.

1. After applying lubricant, pump blood up into the head of your penis with one hand's worth of fingers. The pressure that is produced should be kept for approximately 10 seconds before being released.
2. If you like, squeeze the shaft while doing the motion to increase the amount of blood in the head of your penis.
3. After a little moment of respite, release the squeeze and repeat. While you are free to repeat this as much as you wish, you shouldn't do it for more than 10 minutes at a time.

This activity will eventually increase the capacity of the head of your penis, allowing it to take in more blood. Your penis' end will take on a bell shape as a result.

Developing Width, Option Five

Only your final girth workout option allows you to perform it without lubrication. If you have five minutes to spare and the lubricant bottle is out of reach, this can be useful. Some guys claim that it's also the ideal method to employ in the mornings, right after you awaken from a night's sleep. Many contend that this is the best time to focus on improving your penis because it can be done while you're still in bed without making a mess and it coincides with when your testosterone levels are at their highest during the day.

Simply perform the dry milking technique by carrying out the first or second workout option's instructions. However, since you won't be applying lubricant this time, you won't want to repeatedly run your fingers over your skin. Instead, pull and compress the skin of your penis while avoiding sliding.

If the area is too large to be covered in a single motion, you might choose to work on the base of your penis first, followed by the head end. If you start to feel sore, stop doing the exercise right away and wait at least a day before starting again.

Penis Control: Introducing Kegel Exercises

A larger and thicker penis is all very well, but enhancing your penis has another vital element. By strengthening your Kegel muscle, you will be able to maintain much more powerful erections for a longer time. It will also increase the intensity of your orgasms, and some men even report that they find themselves able to achieve multiple orgasms after working on this muscle for a while. That's not all, either. You will also increase the control that you have over your ejaculations and decrease the amount of time it takes to recover between orgasms. Kegel exercises can even improve the health of your prostate.

The Kegel muscle is actually another name for the pubic-coccygeal muscles, a group that runs from your pubic bone all the way around to your tail bone. If you

want to feel it, press the area just behind your testicles. This is the muscle that controls your urination, but it's also the one that brings you to orgasm and causes your ejaculation to pump. It's present in both men and women, and it's possible you've experienced the pleasure it can bring before—if your partner has ever rubbed this area during a blow or hand job, or even during sex, you will have noticed just how intense the results can be.

It's called the Kegel region because the exercises to strengthen these muscles were named after a gynecologist by the name of Arnold Kegel, who worked out how they

could be strengthened and the advantages of doing so way back in the 1950s. He discovered that contracting the muscles in a controlled way would improve them, just as lifting weights increases the size and strength of your pecs and biceps.

Women have been taught this secret for years and know that it's the best possible way to enhance their sexual pleasure, but for men, it's much less common to even be aware of the Kegel muscles, let alone know how to strengthen them. Ironically, locating the muscle in question and performing

Exercises to strengthen it are actually a lot easier for men. In the next couple of chapters, we'll show you how to find it, and then we'll explain how best to use it—and with these exercises, you'll notice the difference in mere days.

Penis Control: Locating Your Kegels

The first step in improving your penis control is, of course, locating your Kegel muscle in the first place. Once you know where it is and how it feels to flex and release it, you'll be able to do so consciously.

Next time you visit the little boy's room, stop your urine in the middle of the stream. That muscle you can feel straining to hold it back? That's your Kegel muscle.

Now release the stream for a couple of seconds and repeat the exercise. Notice how easily you can stop the flow completely. At first, you might not be able to stop it at all and, at most, you can cause the flow to lessen a little bit. As you exercise the muscle, however, your ability to stop the urine midstream will improve incrementally until, eventually, you can pretty much hold it completely for as long as long as you like.

Stopping your urination is not just a good way to locate the muscle as it happens. It's also the easiest way to regularly exercise your Kegels. Get in the habit of stopping and starting your urine during every single bathroom trip. Try to do so at least five times and gradually lengthen the time you can hold it for.

Count the number of seconds you can hold it for each time and watch as this improves. How tightly you can clench it will also get better, and you should do so.

time to be able to cease your urine flow entirely.

This is a trick that women have been taking advantage of for many years. Some women claim they can hold that muscle in place almost indefinitely, and there's little reason for you to not achieve the same level of strength.

You can also try flexing it quickly and regularly. Especially at first, this can be easier to do than simply holding the muscle tight for an extended time.

Penis Control: Kegel Exercises

Exercising your Kegels does not need to be restricted to your bathroom trips.

Unlike your work to expand the length and girth of your penis, exercising this muscle can be done at any time and in any place. Nobody can see what you are doing, so you can even work on your exercises while you're sitting at your desk or traveling by train.

There are few moments of the day when you won't be able to work on your Kegel muscle, should you decide you want to. It's important to exercise it regularly, so you should try to do at least one set of these exercises every single day. You can vary the type of exercise you do as much as you like, as long as you are working on your Kegels in some manner every day. Here are some options for you to choose from:

contract and release the muscle in a controlled manner, fairly quickly.

Start by doing this for a set of 20 contractions at first, but then begin to build up the number. Eventually, you should be able to do at least 100 in a single session; some men can do 250 at once. For the best possible results, work up to being able to perform a total of 1000 contractions each and every day.

Contract the muscle and hold it in place for as long as you can manage. At first, this may only be for a few short seconds. As you practice, you should be able to build up to holding the muscle in place for 30 seconds or more, which will increase its strength and endurance.

Flex your Kegel muscle for two seconds and then release it. Repeat this as many times as you can, building up the number of times you can do it in a single session.

Flex your muscle to its full tautness as slowly as you can possibly manage and then immediately let go. As you improve at this technique, you will notice that your muscles flutter as you let go of the tension, which can feel

great in itself. Push the muscle outwards, just as you do when you are squeezing the final drops out after urinating. This exercise is best avoided when you need the bathroom, as it can actually squeeze out urine and can also

cause your anus to open—as you can imagine, that can be problematic if you're not paying attention to your timing.

As your muscles improve in health and strength, you will notice plenty of changes in your sexual enjoyment—but there are some changes that you won't notice right away. You'll thank yourself for those later, though. Your

Kegel muscles can help you sustain erections longer even when you're having trouble doing so at all—many doctors prescribe these exercises for erection problems.

These exercises will increase your arousal, prolong and enhance your orgasms, and lengthen how long you last during sex. And later in life, as your body ages, it can help you avoid incontinence because your muscles will still be firm and tight. Combine this with the possibility of multiple orgasms and the ability to delay your ejaculation, and you'll soon be wondering why you didn't start these exercises years ago.

Wrapping Up

When it comes to your penile development regimen, the conclusion is just as crucial as the beginning. Once you've finished your workouts, you should

To prevent negative effects in the long run, give this most delicate area some love and attention.

Start the last stage by giving your penis a light massage to get the blood flow back to normal and work out any kinks. Although the real work in this procedure has already been done, you can purchase enlargement lotions with herbal, natural ingredients for a smoother massage if you so desire.

Apply a hot compress that is comparable to the one you used to begin your fitness regimen next. If you unintentionally harm your cells, this will encourage them to repair themselves; if not, it will encourage relaxation and the formation of new cells.

After thoroughly drying off, you are prepared to get on with your day, secure in the knowledge that you have made a significant advancement toward a healthier, larger, and more potent penis.

The Three Cs: cringe, cry, cry

You may have read this book up to this point anticipating that it would discuss the surgical techniques and equipment that are frequently claimed to have a significant impact on the size of your package. Although most of them are unneeded, a few of them are noteworthy, so we'll look at them in this chapter.

You might feel tempted to speed up the effects with one of the methods you've heard marketed if you started your regimen in search of speedy results and simply can't wait a few months for your fitness regimen to take effect. But should you?

Surgical Techniques:

We would never, ever advise you to spend your hard-earned money on a penile enlargement treatment. In addition to the fact that the extra they add will be wholly insensitive and have no positive effect on your sexual life, there are numerous other things that could go disastrously wrong. Do you really want to sacrifice your favorite body part's health and wellbeing for a few additional inches? There are a number of surgical procedures available, and while they all seem amazing at first, you'll almost certainly change your mind after speaking with a doctor. Studies show that after being fully and accurately informed of the procedure's results, risks, and potential consequences, the majority of men had no desire to proceed with surgery. A tiny penis is preferable to having none at all.

genital pumps You've probably seen all different sizes and shapes of this equipment, some with manual pumps and some with motors. The overall plan is to suck blood into the shaft of your penis to partially suction it, causing it to engorge. The pressure inside the blood vessels rises as the vacuum does. Unfortunately, research has revealed that penis pumps are not only ineffective but also extremely harmful. A study involving over 40 males over six months revealed a cumulative rise of hardly a millimeter. Some men asserted that they were happy with their progress, but this was attributed to the placebo effect and not to a genuine physical improvement.

In certain circumstances, such as when used in conjunction with a tourniquet ring to help a man with impotence have an erection or to cure Peronei's disease,

which causes the penis to curve and shrink, penis pumps can have noticeable good results. It's unlikely to have much of an impact on the average male with an average penis, though. One that has been used for too long may rupture blood vessels, develop blisters, and generally make you wish you had left it in its packaging.

Men sometimes engage in a risky and painful handmade practice known as "clamping." By tightly squeezing the base for a long time to prevent blood from draining back out of it, clamping aims to expand the size of your penis. You already know how uncomfortable an experience this is going to be in your crotch area if you've ever sat on your hand for too long and experienced numbness and pins and needles. Cable clamps, shoe strings, and cock rings are some of the most frequently used tools, all of which are quite risky, especially the last one. It may become very difficult to remove if a metal device is used to trap blood in the penis.

It may be necessary to amputate your penis if the ring cannot be sawed off. And even if the damage isn't quite as severe, clamping usually has long-lasting detrimental repercussions.

Popping Pills:

There is scant evidence that any of the dietary supplements on the market have any impact on penis

growth. We don't advise taking medications that can disrupt the equilibrium of your body, especially if they aren't likely to result in the penile growth you're hoping for. Since the majority of these pills for increasing libido are made of herbs rather than chemicals, they are safer than their equivalents from 20 years ago. If you want to add these substances to your fitness regimen, by all means, go ahead. However, we're ready to lay money on the fact that the benefits you're experiencing have more to do with your routine than they do with the herbs.

The Tiny Weightlifter Men who believed they could make significant gains by strapping weights on their penises have been the subject of horror stories. Any body part that has a brick hanging from it will inevitably extend over time, but the experience won't be enjoyable. Even if you succeed, it's doubtful that you'll still be as sensitive once you're done, and there will be lots of unpleasant consequences if you fail.

In general, if you want to maintain your health and keep your penis in the best possible condition, we advise against using any of these methods. Continue with the workouts; you'll be glad you did.

Adapting your way of life

You might be surprised to find a chapter on lifestyle modifications in a book about penis development, but if you want to succeed, it's crucial that you make a few changes to your diet and daily schedule. Even if you have doubts about a stem of broccoli's potential to expand your package, keep in mind that a healthy body with plenty of energy will be able to use the improvements you make as a result of your exercise routine. What possibly could you stand to lose?

To begin with, there are a few items you ought to eat regularly, making sure to consume at least one serving each day. These meals include:

- *Milk*
- *The sweet potato*
- *Salmon*
- *Tuna*
- *Eggs with broccoli and liver*
- *Bananas*
- *Onions*

Why? Considering that the majority of these foods contain vasodilators, which have the effect of relaxing the blood vessel walls' muscles, your blood flow in that area has an impact on penis enhancement and the power of your erections in general, so it's wise to choose foods that can be beneficial. These foods on their own might somewhat enhance the size of your penis, but not much. The main purpose of eating them is to increase the impact of the exercises you are performing.

Your preferred diet during a penile enhancement regimen is salmon, in particular.

It contains a lot of necessary fatty acids, such as omega 3. To help you produce powerful and long-lasting erections, they thin your blood and improve circulation.

Similar to garlic, onions increase blood circulation, increasing the amount of blood and oxygen flowing into your penis at just the right time.

Every man who has ever added inches to his penis eats bananas as a crucial component of his diet. According to studies, because of the potassium in this fruit, you can successfully enhance your penis while maintaining a healthy heart potassium in this fruit, you can successfully enhance your penis while maintaining a healthy heart. They will also lower your body's salt levels, improving your heart health even further.

In general, choose foods that will increase blood flow so that you can get stronger erections for a longer period of time. Choose lean meats, fresh produce, whole grains, and lean meats instead of processed junk food.

You might also think about ingesting some herbs as teas, pills, or tinctures. Each will contribute to the success of your program and have a good effect on its own.

Extract from Muira Pauma Bark: This herb, which was found by Brazilian Amazonian shamans, stimulates arousal and combats tiredness. Additionally, it eases the corpora cavernosa, which improves your penis' capacity to engorge.

Another herb from Brazil, catuaba bark extract is well known for its capacity to induce a profound state of relaxation while also enhancing your peripheral circulation and sexual prowess.

Hawthorn Berry: This small tree holds a hidden secret that can help you prolong erections and improve penis sensitivity. It will have both short- and long-term benefits that will benefit your penile development program. Because it has a very high concentration of bioflavonoids, hawthorn berries have been used for a long time to cure irregular heartbeats and soften arteries. In order to stimulate more blood to flow through your blood vessels, it is crucial to strengthen your blood vessels. Tongkat Ali'sThis herb genuinely aids in growing the size of your penis as well as your testosterone levels. It increases the size of the cells in your testicles, as well as the size of your penis and the quantity of sperm in your body. It's arguably the most well-known herb for enlarging the

penis, and it's wonderful to include in your enhancement regimen.

Keep in mind that changing your diet alone won't make your penis bigger, and adding herbs or pills won't make a difference that will last.

However, incorporating them into a comprehensive routine will enhance the results of the activities you are performing. Sleep a lot so that your penis has enough time to become firm and saturate itself with the oxygen it requires in the interim. You will experience effects far more quickly as a result of all of these factors working together.

Speed Training

Even though there aren't always enough hours in the day to dedicate to your penile enhancement program, frequent participation will help your results progress more quickly. your exercises. There is an alternative you can attempt in place of regular workouts on days when you are too busy, distracted, or just exhausted to focus on them.

When you don't have time for a full set of exercises, it's not advisable to use a speed workout as your only penile enhancement technique, but there's absolutely little harm in incorporating it into your entire program. It will at the very least assist you in maintaining the advancement you have already made. Even without using other methods, some men report that it has, at most, lengthened their penis by over an inch in a matter of months.

For this one, you might want to start by lubricating your penis, but even if you've just returned from a five-minute bathroom break at work and are without any lubricant, you can still finish the exercise.

1. While seated comfortably, make a circle with your thumb and forefinger wrapped around the base of your penis.
2. Stroke your penis vigorously from the base to the top. Keep your hold as tight as you can without hurting yourself, and do your best to spread the skin as you go.
3. Restart at the base when you get to the end. Repeat the action as necessary, tightening your squeeze a little bit each time. The blood will be confined to your penis as a result. Every time you iterate, speed up.

4. At some point, you will unavoidably feel your penis start to erect. Allow it to continue doing so until you reach full hardness.
5. Retrace your steps to the base and grasp it firmly in one hand. With both hands, extend your penis as far as you can without inflicting discomfort, creating a comparable grasp at the other end, toward the tip.
6. Move your penis to the right and maintain that position for 10 seconds.
7. Straighten your penis and hold it there for another 10 seconds.
8. Move your penis to the left and hold it there for another 10 seconds.
9. Push it down and hold it there for 10 seconds.

After completing all four of the preceding stages, let go of the base of your penis. You will immediately feel the blood start to flow, and you can ejaculate if necessary.

Even during the busiest weeks, it won't take you more than five minutes out of your day to do a speed workout. The exercise can also be done up to three times in one day. However, be careful not to completely cut off the circulation to your penis while completing this exercise, as it is never a good idea. If you experience any discomfort while using this technique, something is amiss with the way you are doing it. It's crucial to avoid extending too much at once and to always apply lubricant.

Your erectile tissue is the target of this speed workout, which, when done, will stretch the skin and cause tension. This indicates that including a speed workout in your regimen has advantages beyond simply increasing penile length. It will make your skin more elastic and increase the amount of room in the corpora cavernosa, the cavernous chambers of your penis. If you're unsure of how valuable having extra air pockets on hand can be, know this: the more blood you can fill these gaps with, the larger the total bulk of your penis when it is in an erect position. and that alone is penis enlargement.

Bringing everything together

You've tried the exercises out, selected the one you like most, and made sure to heed any safety and health recommendations along the way. There is only one thing left to do once you've narrowed down your penis augmentation regimen to the components you're happy with: put everything together.

We'll demonstrate to you in this chapter how to easily incorporate these exercises into a regular routine. You can modify the program to incorporate the exercises that are convenient for your busy schedule, easy for you to perform, and pain-free. Even better, you may change up your routine and alternate the workouts on a daily, weekly, or monthly basis. Your progress will be more even, and your chances of becoming bored will decrease as you add more variety while still working toward the same general goals.

As you put together your program, remember to:

1. No matter which other workouts you choose to do after this, they are all required. 1. Hot Compress Introduction: 5 minutes Always get your penis ready before you begin.
2. Stretch It Out Exercise: 30 minutes: Start your workout with one of the stretches from the first few chapters.

Depending on the workout you select, you might not want to spend a full 30 minutes on this segment initially, but you should try to increase this with time.

1. *Interval*: 1 minute—whip your penis around lightly no more than 30 times following your first workout. Make sure to cup your testicles in your other hand as you do this to prevent them from flying around and getting damaged.
2. *Working on Width Exercise:* 20 minutes to include a girth-increasing exercise in your routine, select your favorite option from the Working on Width chapters.

Again, begin with less than 20 minutes and gradually increase to the allotted time. Remember that you must complete this section without ejaculating and keep your penis semi-erect at all times.

3. *Penis Control Exercises*: 5 Minutes: At this point in your routine, pick a Kegel exercise and carry it out for at least five minutes.

It is included here in part to complete your program and in part to help you remember that this crucial exercise should be a part of your daily routine. You can go ahead and incorporate your control exercises into other parts of your daily schedule if you wish to conduct more or the same Kegel exercises throughout the day or are confident that you will remember to do them.

Concluding: Spend five minutes applying a hot compress to your penis to repair any damage and restore it to its prior, healthy state. Again, this step is a definite necessity.

These six actions, taken together, provide a healthy regimen that will not only assist you in addressing penile enhancement in whatever way you may choose but also make sure you do so in a healthy manner. The secret is repetition; you'll start to see benefits rather quickly, but you should expect significant results in a few months. At least five full workouts should be completed each week, with the low-impact speed workout being substituted only when absolutely necessary.

You will have a larger and thicker penis, more energy to use it, and a much harder erection after your program has fully matured. What more could you possibly want from your partner?

Monitoring Your Development

Obviously, after all this effort, you'll want to periodically check the length and circumference of your penis to gauge your progress. Without us, however, much as dieters are advised to avoid the scales outside of their weekly check-in, it is preferable to conduct a check no more frequently than once a week. In this manner, you will see more significant changes throughout each measure and will be able to gauge the success of your efforts.

Because that's ultimately what you're interested in, you should also make sure to constantly measure your penis in its completely erect state. According to studies, there is absolutely no relationship between the size of your soft penis and the size of your erection. It's possible that you won't notice the same difference in both states because there is such a difference between a "grower" and a

"shower," and because the amount that your penis grows when it becomes erect can range from almost nothing to four full inches. Focus on the state that matters most instead.

It is preferable to measure while your penis is in the state in which you will be using it because the changes you are striving for should be evident and palpable.

One Last Note About Safety

Although we've touched on this topic numerous times throughout the book, it bears repeating before we send you off to your workout because it is so crucial to your general wellbeing, both sexually and otherwise.

Before beginning each workout, double check that you have read the directions completely. You won't be able to make the enhancement gains you desire if you perform an exercise that calls for lube without any or one that calls for a flaccid penis with an erect one, and at worst, you risk doing long-lasting damage.

Avoid going overboard, too. Growing your penis is not a goal that can be accomplished in a single day; you will need to be persistent and patient over the course of several weeks and months. If you still want to be able to walk in the morning, resist the urge to squeeze an entire year's worth of exercise into one day. It will be worthwhile in the end.

If you're discouraged by the slow outcomes, stay away from damaging alternatives to these activities. You have a greater chance of avoiding the more nefarious penile enlargement offers if you know before you start that you won't be measuring more inches after a week. With a high likelihood of doing irreparable harm, utilizing a machine to suck on your penis, getting an operation, or clamping yourself with metal will not produce greater outcomes than regular exercise.

Finally, keep an eye out for any discomfort or pain you may have during your sessions.

These won't always indicate that you should stop, and the instructions will let you know if it's usual to experience them, but they frequently indicate that you should stop. If you experience pain, you may be performing the exercise incorrectly, or you may have completed more repetitions than are currently comfortable for you. You'll get much better results if you pay attention to your body.

Conclusion

Reading the witchcraft and crazy scientist alternatives that are so easily available in the depths of the internet was starting to really irritate us, so we're thrilled to have delivered the true secrets of penile enhancement to you. These methods will provide you with much better and healthier results than a pump or dubious pill bottle, in our experience after using them ourselves.

With these tips in hand, we hope you'll set out on a path to sexual fulfillment that will make you and your partner truly happy. Your penis will not only be the length you've always desired, but it will also be the size that so many women say is essential to their enjoyment. Your penis will stand tall and proud, and your erections will be stable, powerful, and long-lasting. As you establish and gain control over your penis, you will be able to set the tempo and stay in the bedroom as long as you like.

By the time you start adding inches to the tape measure, you'll be more physically fit, more confident, and more than a bit eager to test the results in real life.

You'll no longer delay talking to the person of your dreams out of concern that they will be put off by the size of your package or underwhelmed by what you can accomplish with it since you'll know you have everything you need to become a bedroom legend.

People frequently assert that size isn't everything, and we somewhat concur with that assertion.

The fact is that size only accounts for a small portion of the total picture and is ineffective in the absence of strength, stamina, and confidence. You must possess the entire package in order to be the complete package, which is now possible thanks to this program.

Monitoring Your Development

Obviously, after all this effort, you'll want to periodically check the length and circumference of your penis to gauge your progress. Without us,

However, much as dieters are advised to avoid the scales outside of their weekly check-in, it is preferable to conduct a check no more frequently than once a week. In this manner, you will see more significant changes throughout each measure and will be able to gauge the success of your efforts.

Because that's ultimately what you're interested in, you should also make sure to constantly measure your penis in

its completely erect state. According to studies, there is exactly no association.

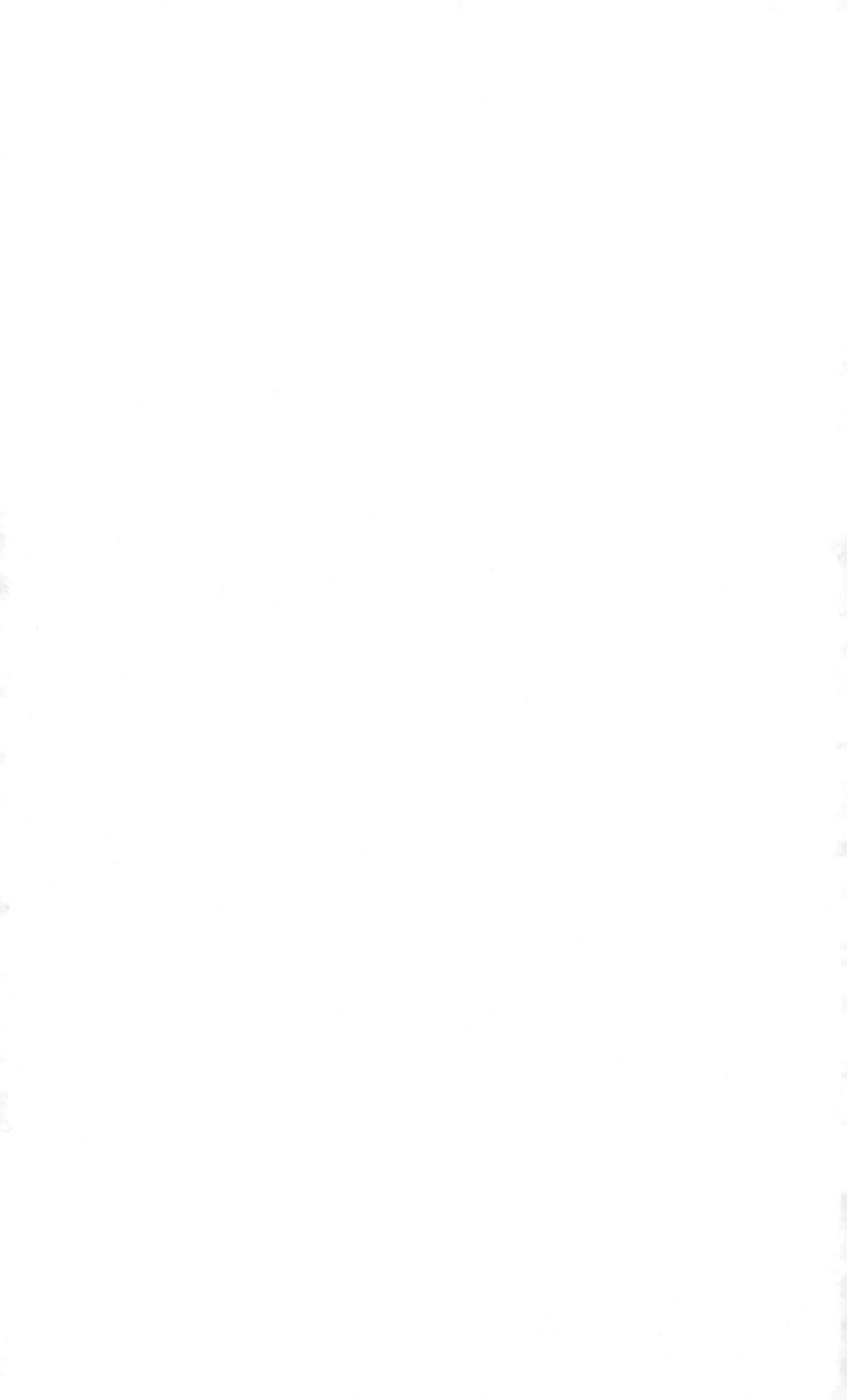